Homemade Lotion 101: A Step-By-Step Guide For Making Your Own Lotion From Scratch

Table of Contents

Introduction

We all need some lotion to keep our skin healthy, moisturized and smooth. There are different varieties of lotions available in the market. Most of them contain ingredients which may harm your body or skin in some way or the other. If you are living in an area where the climate is hot or cold, then you will surely need the lotion to soothe your dry skin. Though the advertisements about the commercial lotion products promise you better looking skin, it is true that they have certain adverse effects on your skin in the long run. Moreover, the branded high quality body lotions are very expensive these days and it is not easily affordable by many people these days. The branded lotions may contain harmful toxins, dyes, preservatives and many other chemicals which may affect the texture and smoothness of your skin when used continuously. It is necessary to use hand lotions on hands only and to use face lotions on face only. Using the hand lotions on the face may cause the pores on the skin of the face to get clogged and it may cause acne and pimples. So, the best option is to go for homemade lotions and with all the ingredients needed to make homemade lotions easily available in the marketplace. Making lotions at home is very easy. The best part about making homemade lotions is that it comes to you at affordable prices and you will find it to be natural and highly cost effective.

Skin Damages

Our skin gets affected by various factors such as: the food we it, the environmental conditions, and continuous exposure to sun, lifestyle, stress, pollution and aging. Poorly nourished skin becomes dry, wrinkled and damaged. Aging also causes dryness and wrinkles in many. People want to maintain their healthy and young skin as long as possible and hence proper caring and nourishment for the skin is a must. The best option to keep your skin healthy and vibrant is to use a homemade body lotion with natural ingredients. It will be totally free from harsh chemicals and also free from preservatives and thereby your skin will always be soft, smooth and clear.

Why Homemade Lotion?

A homemade body lotion is a better choice than the commercial lotion as they have many benefits over the branded or commercial ones. You will be using all the natural ingredients for making the lotion and you will know what the ingredients in the lotion are. This ensures that your skin will be safe after using the lotion. You can create particular lotions to solve the particular skin problems. You can make them in the appropriate consistency you want. You don't have to worry about the greasiness of the commercial lotions. It is very easy to make the body or hand or face lotion at home and you will be able to save lots of money you are spending on ineffective and costly commercial products.

Important Ingredients

The basic ingredients of any homemade lotion are simple and easy to get. The ingredients include water, oil and an appropriate emulsifier. Almond oil, coconut oil and olive oil are good choice of oils to use in lotion as they are non-greasy and light. These oils get easily absorbed by the skin. Bee wax is usually used as the emulsifiers in homemade lotions. You can use purified or distilled water in the lotion.

Benefits Of Using Homemade Lotion

People are going after the homemade body lotions due to the enticing benefits it provides to the body and skin. Following are the major benefits of using homemade moisturizer.

- **You Can Choose The Beneficial Ingredients** - You will be able to decide what all ingredients should be used for making the lotion. You can use the ingredients which suits your skin better. You can use vegan ingredients or natural ingredients for making the lotion. You can add natural and skin nourishing ingredients like cocoa butter, avocado oil, Shea butter, etc. in the lotion.

- **Saving Money** - When you are using natural ingredients, which are easily available for making body lotion, you will be saving lots of money on your lotion expenses. The branded lotions are usually costly because of the cost of the marketing campaigns and overhead cost of the manufacturer.

- **Environment Friendly** - The ingredients used for making the body lotion at home are mostly natural ingredients and are hence biodegradable, the store bought lotions will contain chemicals which are harmful to the environment.

- **You Can Make The Lotions According To Your Skin Type** - If you are preparing the body lotion for particular skin problem, you can choose the right ingredients for it while making the homemade lotion. People with dry skin will need moisturizing substances in the lotion and people with oily skin should use ingredients which will not increase the oiliness of the body.

- **Can Use It In Other Beauty Products** - The homemade skin lotions can be used in making other beauty products such as lip balms and bathing gels. This will improve the quality of the lip balms or other beauty products immensely and will also be free from harsh chemicals and ingredients.

- **It Is Convenient** - You don't have to get appointments from beauty salons and spas to get your skin clean and healthy. You will be saving a lot of time by nourishing your skin at home using the homemade products.

- **Quality And Safe Products -** When you are making the required body lotion at home, you can ensure the quality of the product. You can use quality emulsifiers and aromatherapy oils to make the homemade lotions better in quality.

- **It Makes A Wonderful Gift-** You can gift the homemade lotions to your friends, relatives and colleagues on various occasions. They will appreciate your effort and also the quality of the product. All you need is to prepare the homemade lotions, cover in good looking gift wraps and it becomes a wonderful gift that the receiver will cherish for a long time.

- **It Is Not Time Consuming -** Once you get all the necessary ingredients from the local grocery store or from online stores selling these items, it is simple to make the lotions using the recipes.

- **More Effective –** Since the homemade lotions contain quality ingredients blended in the right ratio, the effects of the lotion will be more than the lotions available in the market. You will be achieving flawless, smooth and vibrant skin using the homemade body lotion.

- **Earning Money** - You can start making homemade lotion as a small business and can earn money at your free time.

- **Solution For Multiple Skin Problems** - Using the different natural you will be able to produce lotions which can cure your various skin problems such as dryness, scars, stretch marks, uneven skin tone, blemishes, acne, oily skin etc.

- **You Can Decide The Scent** - Another advantage of preparing the body lotion at home is that you will be able to select the scents which are well suited for you. You can experiment with different scents every time to get the perfect lotion needed by you.

- **No Need To Worry About Allergies** - Some people may develop allergies when they use the commercial body lotions prepared by using various chemicals and preservatives. Since you will be using natural and skin friendly items in the lotions made at home, you do not have to worry about the risk of skin allergies.

Precautions To Be Taken

When you are planning to prepare the body lotion at home, you should be careful about certain aspects.

- It is important to make sure that you are using a sterilized container to mix the ingredients.

- Always store the lotions in bottles which are sterilized. It is necessary to sterilize the cap as well. When you use unsterilized containers bacteria will start to grow.

- If you are preparing large quantities, or if you want to store the lotion for a long time it is necessary to add some preservatives to prevent the growth of bacteria and mold in it.

- **Keeping Records** - It is better to keep a record of the ingredients used in each lotion and the results achieved by the lotions. This will help you to understand the most effective homemade lotion recipe for your need.

The shelf life of the homemade lotion depends on the ingredients used. Depending on the oil used and the shelf life differs. Some oils become rancid easier than others. The homemade lotions with preservatives added to it will have a shelf life of 6 months. If you do not want to add any preservatives, but want to store the lotion, then you can refrigerate the lotion.

Guide To Make Easy Homemade Lotion

The following are the steps that you need to follow to make the best homemade lotion very easily. You will find doubt that the homemade lotion is as good as any other branded lotions that you can buy in the market if not better. Moreover, you will be able to make the lotion at affordable prices and end up saving a lot of money while shopping cosmetic products.

Ingredients For Homemade Lotion

- ½ cup of oil (coconut oil, jojoba oil, grape seed oil, olive oil, etc)

- 2 to 3 tablespoons of distilled water or aloe vera gel (30 to 45 grams)

- 30 grams or 2 tablespoons of beeswax

- Few drops of essential oils

- Vitamin E oil

Tools Needed

- Measuring cup

- Large sauce pan

- Glass bowl

Step By Step Procedure

1. Keep all the ingredients ready on a table so that you do not have to run around searching for the ingredients and also you can save a lot of time preparing the lotion.

2. The first thing that you need to know is that you can prepare a lot of varieties of homemade lotions with many different oils and ingredients. The basic concoctions needed to make homemade lotions are: distilled water, beeswax, grape seed or coconut oil, few drops of essential oil and vitamin E.

3. Put a saucepan on top of a gas stove and low heat it.

4. Add the grape seed oil or any other oil of your choice, beeswax and vitamin E oil into the saucepan. Mix it and melt them together. You need to prepare this melted mixture with utmost care and slowly. Make sure that you do not burn the materials.

5. If you are heating anything for the first time using a saucepan, then it would be better for

you to try out the double boiling method to melt the ingredients together. All you need to do is to boil water in a saucepan. Pour all the above mentioned ingredients into a bowl that can easily be placed in the boiling water and melt it through the double boiling process. This might take more time than melting it directly. Be patient until the ingredients melt and get mixed properly. This is the best and safe method to melt anything.

6. As soon as the mixture is completely melted, turn off the flame and transfer the melted mixture into a large glass bowl.

7. Now add aloe vera gel or distilled water to this mixture. If you are looking for a thicker and butter like consistency for your homemade lotion, then you need to add lesser amount of distilled water.

8. You need to beat this mixture in a hand mixer or blender so that the lotion becomes thick.

9. You can also substitute distilled water with rose water as it will give a pleasing fragrance to your homemade lotion. Rosewater is easily available in most of the grocery stores.

10.   Now allow this mixture to sit for about 15 to 25 minutes. You can choose to cover the mixture with a cloth or even leave it as it is on the counter top. The mixture will thicken up and congeal in due course of time.

11.   Once the mixture has rested for about 20 minutes, transfer the prepared lotion into a glass jar or a lotion container using a scooper. Your easy and quick homemade lotion is ready to be used.

Full Ingredients

- 22 oz distilled water or aloe vera gel

- 1/2 teaspoon of cinnamon

- 1/2 teaspoon of citric acid

- 1/2 teaspoon potassium sorbate (optional)

- 1 tea bag of your choice

- 5 oz scented oil

- 1 teaspoon (5 g) honey

- 5 tablespoons emulsifying wax or shredded beeswax

- 1 tablespoon (15 g) stearic acid

- 1 teaspoon (5 g) each of selected herbs

- 1/8 teaspoon or dash of vitamin E oil or rosemary extract

Step By Step Procedure

1. It is first important for you to gather all the required ingredients and the tool make the homemade lotion on the kitchen counter top table where you are going to prepare the lotion. This will save a lot of your time and you also do not need to run around searching for ingredients in the middle of the lotion preparation process.

2. In a deep bottom saucepan, add distilled water or aloe vera gel. Now heat the pan on high until the water or the gel begins to boil.

3. Once you spot the bubbles to develop on the water or the gel, reduce the heat from high to medium.

4. Now is the time to add cinnamon, potassium sorbate and citric acid to the boiling water or gel and mixing it well.

5. Once you find that all the ingredients have dissolved in the water or the gel, add a teaspoon of your favorite hers that you have chosen. You also need to dip a teabag of your choice in the water or the gel that is on medium flame.

6. Now simmer all these ingredients in the gel or water for about 10 minutes on medium flame and then reduce the heat from medium to low. Allow the mixture to simmer on low heat for about 30 minutes.

7. In another small pot or saucepan, add 5 oz of the chosen oil (coconut or jojoba or olive or walnut) along with 5 tablespoons of shredded beeswax or emulsifying wax.

8. If you do not have stearic acid, then you need to add 6 tablespoons of shredded beeswax or emulsifying wax.

9. If you have stearic acid, then you need to add a tablespoon of the acid along with your shredded beeswax into the saucepan or pot. If you want your homemade lotion to be a thick one, then you need to add two tablespoons of stearic acid.

10. Now add a teaspoon of organic honey and 1/8th teaspoon of Vitamin E oil or rosemary extract to add more flavor to your homemade lotion. Mix all these ingredients well and leave it aside.

11.   Now in another medium sized pot or saucepan, add water and start to boil the water.

12.   When the water is getting boiled, you can strain all the earlier simmered herb mixture into a large mixing bowl. Make sure that squeeze the herbs as well as the tea bag properly so that all the good juices of the herbs and tea bags are collected in the mixing bowl. It is important for you to use a large mixing bowl as you will be transferring all the ingredients and mixture into this large mixing bowl.

13.   Once the water in the saucepan starts to boil, you need to immerse the pot containing the oils in the boiling water in such a way that you can easily melt the wax and the oils through the double boiling process.

14.   It is very important for you to stir the wax and the oils consistently so that the wax completely dissolves and that it is not overcooked.

15.   Make sure that the oil does not get too hot and remove it from the boiling water sauce pan once you find that all the shredded beeswax has melted nicely. The most important

thing that you need to follow here is that you should not shift your eyes when double boiling the wax and that you should keep on stirring the wax continuously until it completely melts.

16.   You can slightly cool down the mixtures (herb mixture and the wax mixture). But make sure that it does not cool down fully and you need to mix these two mixtures together when it is slightly hot.

17.   You need to beat the herb mixture when adding the oil mixture to it little by little. It is important for you to not add all the wax mixture to the herb mixture and whisk it. You need to blend them together for about two minutes.

18.   You need to continuously whisk and mix the ingredients together so that the mixture is totally devoid of air bubbles. You can add a drop of essential oil or any favorite fragrance to the mixture and the ratio of the fragrance oil to the total mixture will be in the ratio of one drop to 2 ounces of mixture.

19.   The mixture will be a watery one in the beginning and there is nothing to worry about if

your total mixture is watery. You need to give it some time to cool and to set properly.

20.   You need to allow the total mixture to sit for about two to three hours when it will become completely cool and also get thicker.

21.   Once the total mixture has completely cooled down, you can now transfer the mixture into storage bottles. You can use a funnel to easily pour the total mixture contents into the storage bottles. Your homemade lotion is ready.

22.   You can store the homemade solution in the storage bottles and keep it under until you are ready to use the lotion.

23.   The homemade lotion will last for about three months from the date of preparation when kept under normal conditions. Make sure that you do not leave the lotion to get directly exposed to sunlight or hot sun as this will spoil your homemade solution and it will not last longer.

Tips To Prepare Best Homemade Lotions

- It is important for you to make sure that the oil an the herb water mixture is not too hot when mixing and must be having more or less the same temperature while mixing.

- It would be better for you to use aloe vera gel instead of water, as this will help in increasing the longevity of the homemade lotion.

- Adding one percent of honey to the oil content will help in increasing the shelf life of the homemade lotion.

- If you like to get a shiny and greasy look and feel to your homemade lotion, then it would be ideal for you to add about 40 to 50% oil to your lotion.

- It is important to use 0.5 percent of Vitamin E oil to your oil mixture when preparing homemade lotion as it will help in keeping the oil from turning yellow or going stale in your homemade lotion.

- Make sure that the herbs that you infuse in the oil mixture stays on simmer for at least three hours. If you are infusing the herbs into the water, you need to allow them to simmer for a minimum of 35 to 45 minutes.

- Oil and wax ratio must always be 1 tbsp emulsifier or wax for one ounce of oil.

- Stearic acids, lecithin powders or xanthan gums are the main ingredients that you would need if you are looking to thicken your homemade lotion. It has to be added at 1 or 2 percent in the lotion. They must be added to the oil mixture and mix well until they get dissolved in the oil.

- It is important for you to make sure that the homemade lotion is at room temperature before transferring it into the airtight storage containers.

- It is better to use cinnamon powder when preparing homemade lotion. Use of cinnamon oil can cause irritation and allergies to your skin.

- It is important for you to make sure that you do not add any toxic ingredients when preparing homemade lotions. They can easily harm your skin and they can enter straight into your skin, bloodstream and cells.

- It is important for you to not microwave the oil or the water mixture as the molecular structure of the ingredients will change when you microwave. It would turn out to be non beneficial for the skin.

- The most important thing that you need to take care of is to test the homemade lotion on a small area of your body before applying it to your whole body. This will help you to check if your skin is allergic to any of the ingredients used in the preparation of homemade lotion.

www.ingramcontent.com/pod-product-compliance
Lightning Source LLC
Chambersburg PA
CBHW061952280526
45787CB00004B/1823